Overcome Sugar Addiction

Sugar Smart Diet

By Cathy Wilson
Copyright © 2014

Income Disclaimer

This book contains business strategies marketing methods and other business advice that, regardless of my own results and experience, may not produce the same results (or any results) for you. I make absolutely no guarantee, expressed or implied, that by following the advice below you will make any money or improve current profits, as there are several factors and variables that come into play regarding any given business.

Primarily, results will depend on the nature of the product or business model, the conditions of the marketplace, the experience of the individual, and situations and elements that are beyond your control.

As with any business endeavor, you assume all risk related to investment and money based on your own discretion and at your own potential expense.

Liability Disclaimer

By reading this book, you assume all risks associated with using the advice given below, with a full understanding that you, solely, are responsible for anything that may occur as a result of putting this information into action in any way, and regardless of your interpretation of the advice.

You further agree that our company cannot be held responsible in any way for the success or failure of your business as a result of the information presented in this book. It is your responsibility to conduct your own due diligence regarding the safe and successful operation of your business if you intend to apply any of our information in any way to your business operations.

Terms of Use

You are given a non-transferable, "personal use" license to this book. You cannot distribute it or share it with other individuals.

Also, there are no resale rights or private label rights granted when purchasing this book. In other words, it's for your own personal use only.

Overcome Sugar Addiction

Sugar Smart Diet

By Cathy Wilson

Table of Contents

Introduction

"Would you like a little brown sugar on your oatmeal?" A prime example of how society in genera has taken added sweetness to the extreme. Stop for a minute and ask yourself if oatmeal really does need added sugar? Perhaps you could add a handful of antioxidant rich berries or a 1/4 cup of heart healthy nuts and seeds to add more flavor. Or, how about this for a concept, why not teach your taste buds to crave oatmeal completely naked?

I don't mean you get naked, but rather eating oatmeal without anything added what-so-ever. A though if you want to do that and eat it naked that's completely up to you.

We are creatures of habit and most of our poor eating habits are learned. This means over time you have learned to add sugar to your frosted flakes, chocolate chips to your pancakes, and sweet royal icing to your cupcakes.

We condition ourselves to add sugar and expect it, and recognize it's missing if we happen to run out or forget. What's more is sugar is addictive in nature, where your mind and body are going to crave additional every time you have it.

Research shows the spike in blood glucose levels gives you a temporary feel good feeling similar to a runner's high, where your endorphins kick in boosting your energy and triggering that addictive "feel good" feeling.

9

The problem is with a sugar high, you quickly come crashing down to a depressing low, which doesn't happen with an exercise high.

Sugar eating is cyclical in nature, a roller coaster of highs and lows that get higher and lower over time. This triggers emotional eating, interferes with quality sleep, steals energy, gets you fat and lazy, and increases the risk of serious disease that's often preventable.

The Cycle:

Eat Sugar
Get Connected Chemically and Emotionally
Eat More Sugar
Want More Sugar
Becomes Habitual Over Time
Dependency Increases
More Sugar is required to Satiate Cravings
Eat More Sugar

This vicious cycle of sugar induced highs and lows takes control of your life and often interferes with things like going out with friends, work, and even personal commitments. I'm sure you've heard the term "closet eater," this happens when sugars gets a hold of someone and they are embarrassed, ashamed, and even afraid of what the future holds, doing whatever it takes to keep their secret engaged.

In this introductory book you are going to better understand what progress has done to sugar, what sugar is in basic, how to get sugar off your menu, and all the gains you can look forward to when sugar is managed in your life.

Time for you to open your mind and get set to under-standing the nasty of sugar.

Chapter One - Histories of Sugar - The Scientific Perspective

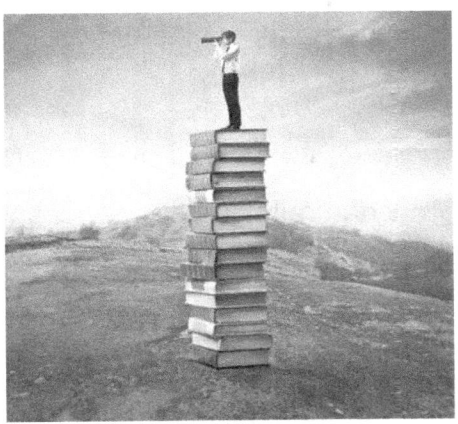

Live Science estimates the average American devour up to 100 pounds of sugar each year. You're living in Fantasy Land if you think that's not going to have consequences. This sweet and addictive additive causes obesity, triggers tooth decay, fuels cancer cells, and will slowly but surely strengthen the free radicals within your body to create and infest you with serious disease.

Everybody and everything has a story, the introduction of sugar into our world is no different.

Basic History of the Sweet Stuff

Coined "White Gold," sugar was the catalyst guiding zillions of Africans over to America around the beginning of the 16th century. It was the deliciously addictive sugar cane of the Caribbean that the Europeans craved, the very beginnings of our world sugar epidemic.

The money made from sugar was so lucrative some experts believe it triggered the divide between Great Britain and America, very powerful.

Sugar Trading

Sugar never grew naturally in the Americas, yet today Brazil boasts the highest production rates. It was the voyage of Christopher Columbus in the late 1400s that brought this sweetness over from the Dominican Republic to Southeast Asia.

At this point many Europeans were already craving sugar, the Spanish "borrowed" from Columbus's sack of sugar and started spreading it wildly throughout the Caribbean. Near the middle of the 16th century, the Portuguese transported it to Brazil, from there it went to the British, French, and Dutch settlements.

In order to increase world production Slaves were shipped across the often treacherous seas, in early 1500, to help grow the sugar plantations steady for the next 300 years. Historically speaking, this was called "The Trade Triangle," where slaves were sent to the New World, and their sweat equity was transported to Europe for profit.

A shocking statistic, by mid-1900, over ten million Africans were forced into slave labor in these Caribbean and Brazil sugar plantations.

Sugar Facts

*1/3 of Europe's economy was from sugar during the 14th, 15th, and 16th centuries.

*An offset was adding rum and molasses to the sugar plantation production, triggering wealth from Jamaica to St. Kitts.

*Historians believe Britain lost its thirteen American colonies because their military man power was so busy protecting their sugar plantation profits.

*After the 7 years of war in 1763, security was set in the West Indies to protect the few sugar plantations Britain still had.

*When the fighting ceased, it was King George III that let some of their sugar plantations in the Caribbean go to France in exchange for a large portion of North America.

SUGAR FACT - It wasn't until the 18th century that cultivation of sugarcane started in the US, and it was in New York City in 1690 that the first refinery was built. It didn't take long for progression to occur, by the end of the century more than 30 factories were up and running.

Did You Know That Sugar Began as a Luxury?

It was used for...

*Sweetener
*Spice

*Medicine
*Preservative
*Treatment for colic

Sugar was VERY expensive up until the mid-1700s.

Sugar transformed with slavery.

Now Sugar is Necessary

Over time, sugar was associated with status and was sought after by everyone. It became commonplace in things like tea and coffee, therefore widely available to the general populous.

The governments saw dollar signs with sugar and heavily promoted it in society. Everyone began wanting more and sugar supply and demand continued to rapidly increase. It quickly transferred over into all sort of foods, increasing the flavor and desire. This triggered a snowball effect and the rest is history!

World Sugar Epidemic?

It isn't really even necessary to have a reputable source tell you that sugar is destroying lives. According to *Bel Marra Health* experts, it's no surprise that sugar is causing serious obesity in America, and shows no signs of letting up.

The sad factor is we are all aware of the dangers of too much sugar, or at least some of them, yet we continue to buy into the sugary based diet that hypnotizes and destroys. Shocking to know that almost all the foods we consume have added sugar; from soda, pop and jams, to cereals, breads, soups, and pastas.

Experts report the average North American consumes approximately 1/2 cup of sugar EVERY DAY! Are you kidding me? The body is not made to withstand the effects of that much sugar physiologically. Your mind and physical function will be negatively smacked with a continuous intravenous of sugar 24/7.

My Thoughts...

Knowing a little bit about the history of sugar and how it's evolved into the monstrous epidemic often described today, makes it easier for you to implement the changes necessary to get rid of added sugars.

What was once a very infrequent treat, perhaps in sugar water if you were lucky a couple times a year, now consumes us, and it's up to you to learn all you can to fight back.

Your body doesn't need sugar in the quantities we consume, history proves that. If you want your reality to change, it's up to you to TAKE ACTION to make it happen, cuz nobody else is going to do it for you!

Chapter Two - Types of Sugar

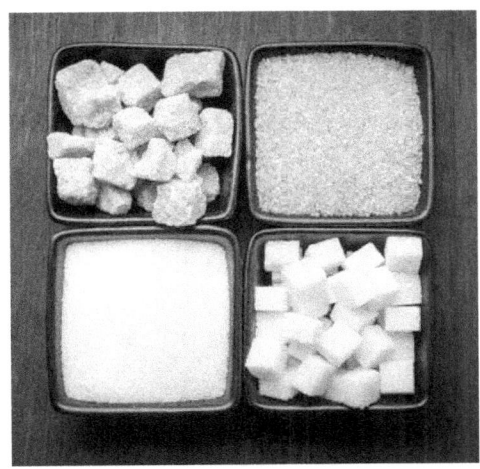

When you're thinking of sugar, I bet the white granular kind comes to mind. It's what you put in your coffee, add to cereal, use for baking, and maybe even sprinkle on your morning fruit. What many don't realize is the capacity to which sugar is present in so many of the foods we eat, in all different types and forms.

Basic white sugar is called sucrose, it is derived from sugarcane or sugar beets.

Did you know that sugar is found in every type of plant, often with fructose and glucose?

The fructose and glucose just aren't in sufficient amounts to warrant manufacturing.

Sugar Types

Xylose - in straw

Maltose - in barley

Sucrose - in plants (glucose and fructose)

Fructose - in sweet honey and fruit

Lactose - in milk and milk products

Glucose - in veggies, fruits, and honey

Galactose - in dairy products

Sugar can be Found Naturally in...

-honey
-beets
-cane
-coconuts
-dates
-maple syrup

*Molasses is a by-product of sugar.

Forms of Simple Sugar - Sucrose

Caster - little bit bigger crystals than icing

Icing - these are tiny small crystals that dissolve quickly in liquid, often used for decorating cakes and pastries

Preserving - large molecules of coarse sugar

Granulated - this is the table sugar we all know and love, with bigger crystals than icing or caster

Bakers Sugar - This specialty sugar is finer than fruit sugar and was created by the baking industry for specialty recipes

Coarse Sugar - Typically known as pear or decorating sugar, it's recovered when molasses-rich sugars crystallize, they are resistant to structural change

Date Sugar - This sugar is high in fiber, doesn't dissolve in liquid, and is made from ground up dates and rather pricey

Fruit Sugar - Smaller than regular sugar, it often comes in pudding mixes and powdered drinks

Maple Sugar - Derived by heating maple syrup to about 50 degrees F, let it cool down to about 200 degrees F, stirring it until it becomes granular

Ultra-Fine Sugar - This is the finest of all white sugars, great for meringue pies and sweetening drinks because it dissolves easily in liquids

Brown Sugar

Light and Dark Brown Sugar - Molasses flavors this sugar that's often used for making butterscotch and glazes, it's rich unique flavor also makes it excellent for gingerbread and baked beans

Muscovado Sugar - A British brown sugar with a deep molasses taste, it's stickier than normal brown sugar

Demerara Sugar - It's light brown with big golden crystals, a hit in England it's often used in after tea

Turbinado Sugar - A partially processed raw sugar, with just the surface of molasses washed off, leaving it with a mild flavor and color

Free Flowing Brown Sugars - A co-crystallization process makes these sugars with powdery finish, not as much moisture as normal brown sugar

Liquid Sugar

Invert Sugar - Where the sucrose is split into two, fructose and glucose, its liquid in form, sweeter than sugar, and often used by food manufacturers

Liquid Sugars - Essentially this is white sugar dissolved in water before use, often used for baking

Red Flag - "Fake" High-Fructose Corn Syrup

High fructose corn syrup is hugely controversial in the medical world, with a reputation for being fattening and unhealthy. It's not derived from plants but rather corn, establishing presence in the early 60s in sodas and processed foods because it's cheaper than real sugar.

Many scientific studies have been done concluding that HFCS is the leading cause of obesity in America. That's a huge generalization, but many experts in the field of health and wellness stand strong with this belief.

What is HFCS?

High fructose corn syrup provides calories to sweeten drinks and foods, often the processed kind. Essentially, it's made through an enzymatic process from glucose syrup that comes from corn. It's fairly new in our food scene and was founded in Japan in the late 60s. It wasn't until the early 70s it found its way into the American diet.

Why do manufacturers love it?

*It's sweeter than sugar
*Mixes well with other foods
*Is cheaper than regular sugar
*Works well in maintaining a longer shelf life for food

What foods typically have HFCS?

*Sodas
*Salad dressings
*Ice-cream
*Cakes and pastries
*Muffins
*Sauces
*Jam

The two kinds of high fructose corn syrup in the market today are HFCS-55, used in soft drinks, and HFCS-42, used for ice-cream, fruit syrup, and baked goods, both are made of different percentages of fructose and glucose.

What's the difference between table sugar and HFCS?

Both are made of fructose and glucose, out with table sugar they are chemically bonded together, so the body has to work to break the bonds down before digesting. With high fructose corn syrup these bonds are just blended together, meaning digesting isn't required to get energy into the blood stream.

Some experts believe this unnatural process causes issues with blood sugar stability and interferes with optimal body function. Think of it as lazy man's sugar, not to mention the fact it's fake and may trigger chemical confusion. Ultimately, it's not a natural substance in this form and therefore might well be considered toxic by the body.

Faster absorption into the blood stream may lead to obesity in American, that's what some of the experts are concluding anyway.

Does HFCS make people fat?

A controversial subject as you know. What the AMA, American Medical Association has found is, although suspicious, there isn't concrete evidence to prove HFCS is any worse than an excess of table sugar.

Bottom line is too much of anything is not a good thing.

My Thoughts...

Sugar really can be confusing but understanding the differences between different sugars and their purpose is going to help keep the water clear for gaining knowledge on why you need sugar and how much is too much. Next, we'll have a look at hidden sugars and how you can take action to battle and win.

Chapter Three - Where Sugar Hides Out and Why

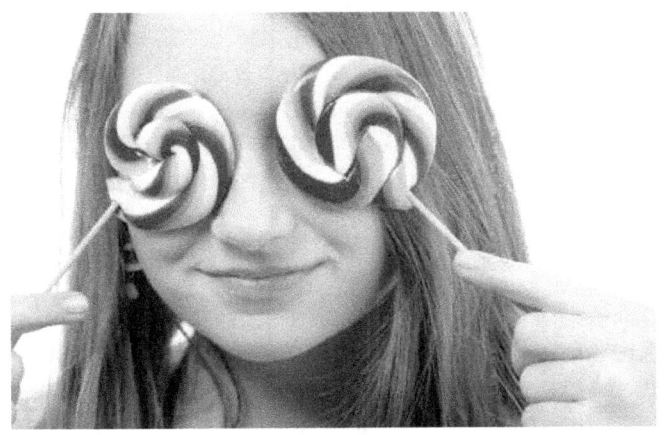

It's much easier to ignore something you know is likely bad for you, but you can't see it so you can sort of just pretend it's not there. I think you know what I'm trying to say. For instance, having a piece of triple chocolate cake is likely going to play the guilt card on you because there's pretty much zero chance of your ignoring the whopping amount of sugar, fat, and calories in it. However, if you were to eat a packaged bran muffin, loaded with harmful sugars and Trans fat, because "bran" is associated with goodness, it will probably be easier for you to feel better about eating it. Sounds silly, but it's very true.

Sad news is, you are likely better off eating the cake and ditching the muffin, this is where the facts and reality get mixed up and often people don't bother figuring it out. Something that makes junk food maker smile big time!

Hidden sugars get us into deep trouble, mind over matter, and when we don't see something we can just pretend it isn't there. Problem is, the end result can't be ignored, which is lots of extra layers of fat, mood swings, health issues like diabetes and circulatory issues, increased bouts of depressions and anxiety, and even serious sleep issues.

Hidden Sugars Hurt!

The AHA reports Americans are getting up to 5 times the sugar they need, and between you and I, that's very conservative. We are conditioned to add sugar to things like tea and coffee, sprinkle it on pancakes, some even add it to popcorn with the butter. With that, you've just taken an okay snack and made it totally bad for you.

Any set problem, is we seem to want more with everything, and this includes sugar. Perhaps we condition our taste buds to like a certain amount of sweetness, get tired of this and soon need a little more to get to that base satisfaction level?

Another issue is even when we are trying to avoid foods loaded with sugar, manufacturers somehow find a way to process foods that have hidden sugars you'd never think were there. So when you are trying to do the right thing, you're set up for failure. That's your reality unless you take charge to make sure you know where those hidden sugars are, so you can choose to "un-learn" them.

You know most of the foods with oodles of sugar; ice-cream, cookies, cakes, pastries, sodas, packed muffins, and so forth. Here are a few foods you might think are angel innocent, but they are devil guilty.

Secret Foods with Sugar

PEANUTS - Be wary that regular mixed nuts and peanut can have added sugar. There are some that don't, but I hate to say most have some extra sugar tossed in.

TOMATO SAUCE - You wouldn't think tomato sauce has sugar, but it's packed. The sugar is used to help take the heat off the acidity. There are varieties that contain less sugar, but you're best to take control and make your own!

SALAMI - Most wouldn't think salami and other deli meats have sugar, but many have this and many other things added in. Check the label before you buy just to be safe.

BAKED BEANS - A totally healthy food, except that it's packed with sugar. Try the all-natural food section in your grocery store to see if you can find some with less sugar.

YOGURT - Everyone loves to grab that little yogurt as they're headed out the door, the flavored ones. Unfortunately, these flavors are topped up with sugar. Again, you need to read the label, smart to buy plain yogurt and add your own fruit to sweeten it.

CANNED SOUP - Bet this one is a surprise! Any condensed, ready to go soup is loaded with sugar. Looks like you might just have to break down and make your own here to avoid all that extra sweet stuff that really isn't necessary.

ENERGY BARS - This could be one of the most misleading sugar buggers around. Strategic marketing for these products makes you think energy bars with all their added protein, are healthy snacks to have regularly. Unfortunately, the majority of energy bars are loaded with added sugar, fat, and calories, and many have very little protein. Some are no better than eating a freakin candy bar. So sad, but so true. Just make sure you read the label before you buy.

WATER and JUICES - Vitamin water is the new thing in the drink world these days, all of which are LOADED with sugar. Juices may draw you in with the "fresh fruit" label, but if you look closer, it's likely 10% juice from concentrate and the rest is sugar.

Just be sure to read the label before buying, and if you see sugar in the first few ingredients mentioned on the list, then you need to drop it and start reading another. Better yet, why don't you just go to the tap and get yourself a nice ice cold glass of water to quench your thirst minus the sugar?

SALAD DRESSINGS and CONDIMENTS - We try so hard to eat healthy, making a salad from scratch, only to ruin your good health intentions by dosing it with fatty sugary salad dressing.

I kid you not, salad dressings are chalk full of sugar, as are most condiments. Try and look for a reduced sugar version or go really easy on them. You do want to eat a salad with a little dressing, not a little salad with your dressing right?

CRACKERS - Most are aware a lot of sugars are found in crackers, but what about the unsweet kind? Truth is, crackers you would think have no sugar, like Triscuit and Ritz crackers, do have sugar added. Makes me sad to break that to you, but it's important you start with the truth and adjust your eating accordingly.

My Thoughts...

If you are serious about reducing your sugar intake you are going to have to get smart. You will have to be on guard against all these hidden sugars found in sneaky foods like low-fat smoothies, whole wheat crackers, and quick to make soups.

This means you're going to have to read the labels of the foods you buy and search for sugar, glucose syrup, corn syrup, sucrose, and all the other fancy names manufacturers try and hide their added sugars behind.

Take action and you will beat the sugar bug!

Chapter Four - Sugar Myths

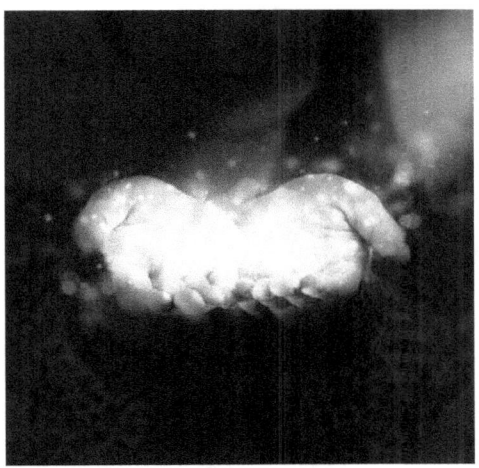

If you think sugar makes you fat, ruins your teeth, and causes your kids to run around like hyper lunatics, you need to read on! Mistruths about sugar often end up interfering in good health because you don't have the factual sugar information you need to make the best decisions for you and your family.

Sugar is something your body needs to survive, but same as everything else it needs to be in moderation. Here are a few myths debunked that are only going to help you get control of your sugar faster.

Mistruth # 1 - Eating sugar will make you a diabetic.

Truth - Sugar itself does not cause diabetes. It's a combination of genetics, poor eating habits, not enough exercise, and not so great lifestyle choices. There is no one causal factor for developing diabetes. However, by eating excessive amounts of the white stuff you will increase your risk of developing diabetes because sugar surges blood glucose levels, the number one factoid in developing diabetes.

Do yourself a favor and prevent diabetes from ever setting in by taking action to reduce your overall sugar intake right now!

Mistruth #2 - If you consume sugar it will make you tubby.

Truth - Sugar is a simple carb, that when eaten in large quantities without exercising, is going to make you fat. What people fail to realize is that eating anything in gynormous amounts over a long period of time will cause weight gain.

Experts say there are approximately 3,500 calories in every pound, which means if you want to lose just one pound of fat you need to take in that number of calories less each day. The most effective way is to combine eating healthier and exercising so that you are burning off more energy and consuming less overall.

Bottom line is that sugar in moderation will not make you fat when included in a healthy lifestyle. If you want to argue further, take it up with the experts.

Mistruth #3 - Filling your kids full of sugar is going to make them totally uncontrollable.

Truth - I always used to believe this one, but according to doctors and other medical professionals in the field, sugar doesn't make your kids hyper. In fact, sugar really makes the body physically sleep in large doses, not spazzy hyper. The excitement is caused by the event itself and not the candy and cake your little one has devoured.

Mistruth # 4 - Careful with sugar because it's addictive.

Truth - The truth here is that no food substance has the physical ability to become addictive. You may crave or desire a certain food for various reasons, but addiction isn't one of them.

What does happen is that sugar dopes up your blood sugar levels, increasing the serotonin in your blood, boosting your pleasure mood temporarily. There are some links this feeling of "food" will sway your mind into thinking it needs more sugar to get to that state again.

Just remember that sugar itself can't be addictive like alcohol or cocaine is.

Mistruth # 5 - There's no nutritional goodness in sugar.

Truth - There's a little bit of a mix-up here. Anything that has calories has nutritional value, therefore sugar does have nutrition. It provides energy so your body can function. Without going further, bottom line s sugar has nutritional value.

Mistruth # 6 - All added sugar is nasty.

33

Truth – Unfortunately, your body can't communicate to you with words what it thinks about added and natural sugars. Experts conclude that sugar is sugar as far as your body is concerned. What many people don't realize is that apples, bananas, and other "natural" foods are loaded with sugars, not just the processed stuff.

Myth # 7 - The food manufacturers are plotting to get us hooked on sugary foods.

Truth - Sure this may run through your mind, but the only person filling your cupboard with sugar just is YOU!

My Thoughts...

People act on the information they have in their brain at the time of the decision. By making sure you have accurate information about sugar and how it affects you and your life, you are going to have the ammo required to reach your health goals without too many unexpected detours.

Here's one example of where the truth doesn't hurt.

Chapter Five - Benefits of Removing Excess Sugar from your Diet

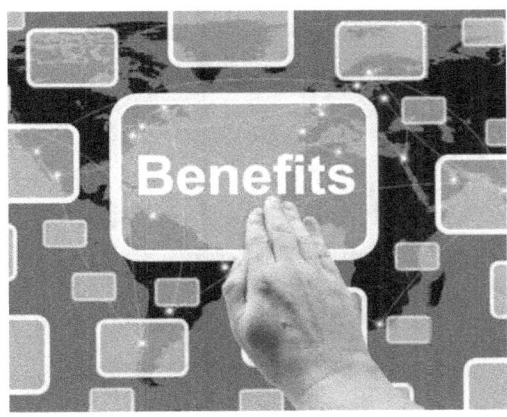

Processed sugars in gynormous amounts are not good for you. In fact, it's likely the unhealthiest ingredient in your diet today. If you don't believe me just ask your mother, sister, brother, doctor, partner, friend, or even the Yahoo behind the donut counter.

Now, it's important to stay reasonable here, you can't ever expect to cut sugar completely out of you daily eating, because it does occur naturally in fruits and veggies, and dairy products. Of course, to cut all these out of your diet would be a pretty Dumbo move.

What most of us need to focus on is added sugars. We need to cut out the sweet crappy food eating and make healthier choices that over time will become habit, our new "normal."

35

Here are a few iron clad reasons to stop and check-in with your extra sugary eating, complements of the big bad world of processed fast foods.

*Very Little Nutritional Value - If you are filling your gas tank mainly with Twinkies, chips, cookies, cakes, frozen dinners, and fast food junk, you are adding in the sugars, fat and calories, and striking out giving your body the good fat, lean protein, complex carbs, and essential vitamins and minerals it requires for optimal health.

Action Step - Choose to avoid processed fast foods, cakes, packaged and boxed foods, and other "junk foods," opting for healthy clean eating. This means choosing lean meats, healthy whole grains, fruits and veggies, beans, lentils and legumes, along with healthy fats instead of the sugary junky stuff.

Stick with it and you will see and feel fantastic!

*Sugars Encourage Fat Deposit in Your Liver - Every time you eat fructose it heads to the liver. If you don't eat fructose after exerting energy, like after a good hike, your body will use glycogen stored in your liver for energy, transforming fructose into fat.

Over time the fatty tissue in your liver will manifest and put you at risk for Non-Alcoholic Liver Disease.

Consistently eating large amounts of fructose is going to fatten up your liver and make you seriously ill.

Action Step - Commit to making better food choices. Eat an apple instead of having apple pie, grilled chicken instead or deep fried, and a bowl of steel cut oats instead of sugary breakfast cereals. The choice is yours.

*It's Sugar that Triggers Insulin Resistance - Insulin is a natural hormone in your body directed glucose out of your blood and into awaiting cells and tissues. When sugar is being abused, this causes insulin resistance, where the cells don't accept the glucose sugars and these sugars concentrate in your blood.

What many don't know is that insulin also dictates to your cells to absorb fat from the bloodstream, while keeping the fat they already have.

You can see how all that sugary junky food interferes with normal insulin production and function, leading to weight gain, ultimately obesity.

Further still, as this insulin resistance progresses, the beta cells in your pancreas getting mucked up and stop making insulin. At this point, you're developed Type 2 Diabetes, affecting over 350 million people globally.

Action Step - Pay attention to the foods you are eating. Look for all-natural whole foods from Mother Nature, and steer clear of packaged and boxed foods that you know are oozing with added sugar, chemicals and preservatives.

*Sugar Triggers Resistance to Leptin - This is a hormone that your fat cells manufacture. Makes sense the more fat you have the more leptin that's in your system. Leptin is meant to signal to your brain that you're full, and to stop eating, along with raising your temperature.

This issue is that the leptin in fat people isn't working, this resistance that has developed from too much sugar is causing interference so the message isn't getting to the brain in time that you're full.

It doesn't help that insulin blocks leptin and fructose raises blood fat, also blocking leptin signals.

All of this makes you think your fat cells are empty and in need of more food, Willpower is no match for blocked leptin messages.

Action Step - In order to reverse this situation you MUST send the sugar packing so leptin and insulin can function properly. This is an all or nothing scenario to the extreme. If you REALLY want to lose fat and get your life back again, you need to cut out all junky sugary foods, and start retraining your brain to crave all the naturally wholesome foods of the earth.

Once again the choice is yours to make.

*Get Control Over Your Weight - 1 gram of sugar has 4 calories of carbohydrate energy. Unhealthy processed foods loaded in sugar also come with oodles of extra bad fat and calories. So by chopping added sugar foods out of your diet, like candy bars, cookies, chips, donuts and soda, you are going to drastically decrease your total daily caloric intake, which will trigger weight loss. Add some effective interval cardio and weight training to your new healthier eating strategy, and the flub is going to disappear faster.

According to the current *Dietary Guidelines of the U.S. Department of Health and Human Services*, added sugars in cookies, pied, donuts, candies, chips, and energy:

*Control Blood Sugars - Avoiding pumping your system full of added sugars is going to help you control your

38

mood, keep energy levels up, deter depression and anxiety, prevent diabetes, and improve your sleep to start. Sugary foods have a high glycemic reading and these simple carbohydrate foods spike your blood glucose levels short term.

This isn't good for physically or mentally.

Action Step - Eating 4-5 healthy mini-meals evenly throughout the day of a portion of protein, complex carbohydrates, and healthy fat, is going to help keep blood glucose levels regular and this will help your internal body function optimally and crisp up your thinking.

For the average female, a sample mini-meal could be a slice of whole grain bread with a tablespoon of peanut butter and an apple, or a small grilled chicken breast with a cup of spinach sprinkled with 1/4 cup slivered almonds, water to drink.

*Better Oral Hygiene - You're not going to get any dentists arguing with your here. Sugars are the cause of cavities and reducing the sugary foods in your diet, while brushing and flossing your teeth twice daily is going to help you reduce cavities and decrease your chances of future dental hygiene issues.

What many fail to recognize is that the health of your gums and teeth correlates with your overall health and wellness. For instance, if you have a bad tooth or infection in your mouth, it's your whole body that's fighting it and this infection is flowing throughout your whole body, not just your mouth.

Good oral health is critically important in your big picture health and wellness plan.

Action Step - See your dentist for regular checkups and choose to eat a diet void of extra sugars. You deserve to be completely healthy, and when you make this decision it WILL happen.

My Thoughts...

By setting a plan out to remove excess sugars from your daily diet, you can see how much improved your overall health will be. It's all about first committing mentally to making the choice to ditch added sugars, and then working to create a master plan that will take you to your goal.

Naturally, this will include healthy "Mother Nature" foods choices, Throw in some regular intense daily exercise including weight training, cardio, core, and stretching exercises, and you are going to blast your health into a whole new orbit that's thinner, stronger, sexier, and happier.

Chapter Six - Pointers on How to Remove Sugar from Your Diet

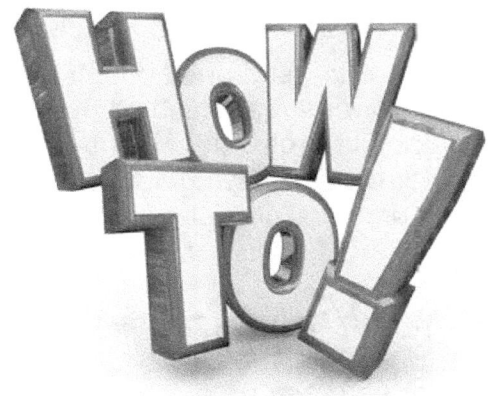

Sugars seems to work on a supply and demand mentality. The more you have, the more you crave, the less you allow yourself, the less you want. It's a give and take relationship and you should be aware that if you are a major sugar addict, it's inevitable you're going to experience some tiredness, grumpiness and perhaps even a few headaches during withdrawal.

Stick with it because it won't take more than a week for the tables to turn and you'll feel fantabulous.

Some choose to jump in with both feet and just prepare themselves to feel off for a few days. Other people like to wean themselves off their usual hamburger and fries, chips, pastry, donut, candy bars, and soda diet. They might start with a couple days of eating healthy each week, then progressing forward from there.

You know your tolerances and preferences and need to act accordingly, so you can set yourself up for success.

If you need help here to get started, inspired, or held accountable to reach your sugar slashing goals, don't hesitate to get a health professional, nutritionist, dietician, or trainer involved. Usually having someone outside your immediate family or social circle is more effective with results.

Pointer One - Whole Grains Replace White

Flip the switch here and get rid of white breads, rice, and pasta, bringing in the healthy whole grain breads, whole wheat pasta, and brown rice. These "brown" food choices are lower on the glycemic index and metabolize slower in your system, offering energy long, along with increased nutrients and fiber.

White bread products are simple sugars that spike blood sugars, shooting your high fast and dropping you to depressing levels faster, while increasing your risk of obesity.

Try one move at a time here. If you usually have two pieces of white bread for breakfast with butter, try one piece of white and one piece of whole grain bread with a smear of peanut butter. When you are ready shift to two pieces of whole grain bread and make this your new normal.

Pointer Two - Keep Your Blood Sugars Up With Regular Mini-Meals

We talked a little about the advantage of fuelling your body with mini-meals already. By always having something healthy in your tummy you are less likely to cave to your sugar craving. Swaying blood sugars are a trigger of junk food eating.

Pointer Three - Discipline in Eating

Did you know that you actually program yourself to crave sweets? One way is by grabbing a candy bar or bag of cookies to tie you over when your tummy in rumbling before dinner. This teaches your body to crave junk when your body is truly hungry.

Next time you are feeling like you've run out of steam, make sure you have a piece of fruit, handful of nuts, or maybe an all-natural yogurt handy. Healthy food to reprogram you to physiologically crave healthy food when hunger strikes.

Pointer Four - Record it

You may snuff your nose at this, but recording the food you eat is a sharp reminder to make the right food choices in the proper amounts for your size, and lifestyle. This will put right in your face how much added sugar you're actually eating. Sure, it may hurt initially, but it does get easier.

Pointer Five - Pay Attention to the Label

You are going to have to read labels if you're serious about finding all those added sugars that are making you fat. It won't take you long to get used to this and it can pretty much predict all the ingredients in the foods you eat.

Pointer Six - Pay Attention to Your Emotions

Emotions and logic physiologically don't mix. When you are depressed, anxious, nervous, or tired, your sugar cravings are more likely to strike. Be prepared and look to gain better control of your emotions. Removing added sugars will to wonders with this. Whatever you do, just don't give up.

Pointer Seven - Craving Junk - Grab Healthy Sweet

Acknowledge when craving a sweet treat, just don't cave, and look to make better choices. If you're itching for a candy bar, try a healthy whole grain granola bar sweetened with honey, or a handful of nuts with raisins. Dried fruit, a piece of fruit, or a slice of whole grain bread with a smear of organic jam works too.

Remember you're not looking to be perfect, just make better decisions for you.

Pointer Eight - Have Access to a Dietician or Nutritionist

Having a nutritionist available is going to help you make the best decisions for you, shortening the time it will take you to kick your sugar eating out the door for good.

Pointer Nine - Quality Sleep Matters

If you commit to getting quality sleep so you are well rested, you're more likely to have on a better head to handle the sugar cravings. Ridding your body of a constant influx of processed sugars is also going to help better your sleep. Research studies show sugar interferes with quality sleep and sleep length. Remove it and you'll be sleeping like a baby soon enough.

Pointer Ten - Chuck it Far!

If you seriously want to get extra sugars out of your body, you're going to have to remove temptation. This means purging your mansion, house, or sugar-shack of all junky sugar foods. It's much tougher to get all sugared up if you don't have candy bars sitting on the table, or donuts hiding in your freezer just in case.

You need to take action here and focus on prevention. The first step in successfully removing sugars is to push them out of your site and surroundings.

My Thoughts...

I'm not sure about you, but I can use all the help I can get to get unnecessary added sugars out of my day, week, and life. We are creatures of habit, which makes them hard to break.

Commit to using the pointers that make sense to you, to help bust up your sugar eating permanently! You are the one calling the shots here.

Chapter Seven - Refocus - The Big Picture

Stop for a minute to ask yourself what your ultimate goal is here. If you are looking to lose 20 pounds permanently, you are going to have to do more than just cut added sugars out of your eating.

In your big picture of fantastico health, you're going to need to consider the foods you eat, exercise routine, mental, emotional, social, health, and lifestyle factors. Each one is reflective of your overall health and wellness, weight, and outlook on life.

Let's have a look at all the pieces to your fantabulous health puzzle. Easing off of the added sugar is just the beginning.

Nutrition

We know sugary foods are high in nutrition-less calories. This means your first step toward great health is to reduce processed fatty sugary high-calorie foods. Avoid Pop tarts, Twinkies, chips, crackers, cookies, brownies, ice-cream, and all those foods you know are NASTY!

Next, you need to start filling your noggin with healthy eating, better food choices than have been making. Start slow, so you don't get overwhelmed and look to eat healthy mini-meals regularly throughout the day.

For simplicity we're going to base the average food servings or amounts on a 2000 calorie diet, something the average moderately active woman might eat to maintain her weight.

Each day she should get...

*2-3 servings of lean protein (lean meat, eggs, beans, quinoa, milk products, and peanut butter)

Serving Sizes - for lean beef and chicken it's about 4-6 oz, the size of your palm; 1 egg;1/2 cup beans; 1/2 cup quinoa; 1/2 cup yogurt, 2x2 inch cube cheese, 1/2 cup yogurt; 1-2 tbsp. peanut butter

Protein Purpose - Next to water, protein is the most abundant substance in your body, with every cell containing protein. Muscles are made of protein so you need to eat plenty of lean protein to build your muscles lean and strong. Proteins also help maintain optimal cell function, help nails and hair grow, and skin to be picture perfect beautiful. Add to this that protein helps maintain and repair cells.

*6-10 servings of complex carbohydrates (healthy whole grain bread, whole wheat pasta, whole grain rice, fruits and veggies)

Serving Sizes - 1 slice of whole grain bread or bagel; 3/4 cup of whole grain pasta; 3/4 cup whole wheat rice; 1 piece of fruit or 3/4 cup fruit salad; 3/4 cup cooked or raw vegetables

Note - If you ever have a rumbling tummy throughout the day, or after one of your mini-meals, have an extra serving of vegetables or fruit. The fiber will fill you up with loads of nutrients and very few calories.

Complex Carbohydrate Purpose - Complex or "good carbs, have 5 main functions:
*Helps control blood sugar levels and produce energy
*Saves the body from breaking down protein muscle for fuel
*Provides the body with fiber
*Prevents ketosis by breaking down fatty acids
*Provides fuel fir the central nervous system

*1-2 servings unsaturated good fats (olive oil, olives, avocado, almond oil, safflower oil)

Serving Sizes - 1-2 tbsp. of unsaturated oil, 3-4 olives, 1/2 cup sliced avocado)

Healthy Fat Purpose - Polyunsaturated, monounsaturated, or healthy fats are necessary for vitamin A, D, E, and

K absorption, which helps with maintaining strong bones and teeth, cell division, maintains body fluid levels, protects vitamin stores, and decreases your risk for serious disease.

Specialty Note Omega 3-6 Fatty Acids - These fatty acids are required a few times a week and are necessary for everything from building cells, to maintaining nerve and brain function. Your body can't manufacture them so you've got to get them from food sources.

Omega-3 is found in fatty fish like salmon, tuna, and mackerel.

Omega-6 is easier to get and found in numerous plant oils like sunflower and corn oil. It's also in various nuts and seeds.

Exercise

Exercise is critical in the big picture of good health. It's also an awesome move to help curb your added sugar habit. Let's say you usually sit down in the early evening to watch a little television with your bag of chips, soda, candy bars and cake or pastry treat.

Your system is used to a standard sugar injection and you need to change it. By picking your butt up off the couch and getting physically active, you're releasing those "happy pill" endorphins that your sugar kick tries to mimic. Instead of spiking your blood glucose levels, you will be pumping up the volume in your heart rate and lung function, purging built up toxins from your system and strengthening your physical body and mental thinking.

This isn't just going to happen if you try it once, and you might not like it the first time. The key is to stick with the pattern until it becomes habit, you accept it and dub it your new healthy normal.

So going for a run and lifting a few weights, swimming, or heading out for an intense hike, where you are coming back with a little sweat on your t-shirt, is going to work wonders with energizing you, reshaping your mind, body, and life perspective beautiful.

The human body was made to move, like it or lump it your body was made to be challenged physically and mentally EVERY DAY, and finger pumping on your electronic devices does not count, nor does all the yapping your do on Skype and your cell.

Fantabulous Excuses to Exercise

*Stabilize your weight. Regular intense cardio and muscle building exercise will help your body to be more forgiving. You have control over the amount of energy you expend exercising. The more you exercise, the more calories you burn.

Life happens and it's important you understand ANY extra physical activity you do counts, whether it's taking the stairs instead of the elevator, or walking four blocks to work instead of driving to the doorstep.

Choose to incorporate effective interval training to blast fat and calories and you will be one step closer to gaining control of your weight, body, and life.

*Fuels energy. By exercising you will strength your physical body, enabling your to feel energized and alive, able and more importantly willing to tackle feats you might have passed by in years past. When you exercise you increase the amount of energizing oxygen that gets to your muscle and vital body organs, this improves performance, so you can do more and will want to accomplish more, and that's amazing.

*Kicks Moods Swings in the butt. By exercising, you are releasing endorphins that you leave feeling on top of the world. Some say these legal chemicals are addictive and I most definitely agree on that one. Getting your heart rate pumping also helps with the psychological of it all, looking better and just knowing you are taking action will boost your confidence and spread your perma-smile a few inches wider.

*Prevents disease. At any level, experts report exercising lowers LDL, bad cholesterol, and boost the good stuff, HDL. It also lowers fats in your blood, helping it to flow with less effort and more efficiently.

*Better sleep. In order for your mind and body to function optimally you need to shut down for at least 7-8 hours a night, according to sleep experts from the *National Sleep Foundation of America*. Studies show regular exercise helps people sleep longer and deeper than couch potatoes.

Just make sure you doing your heart pumping exercise at least 3 hours before bedtime. Too close to when you're hitting the hay will communicate to your body it's time to wake up, not shut down.

*Better Sex. If you ever want a universal excuse to exercise aside from battling sugar eating, it's to heat up the bedroom. Research shows physically active people feel better about themselves, their body and life, and this reflects positively on their need, want and desires to get funky in the bedroom. Exercise also helps improve arousal and for all you gents, reduces the chances of erectile dysfunction. Need I say more?

Getting at least 30 minutes each day of intense physical activity, exercise that makes you sweat and exert some, is going to help you lose or maintain weight, curb sugary food eating, and help you switch your big picture life switch to positive.

Mental/Emotional Considerations

Paying attention to your mental health is essential in making sure you see your big picture positively. It really doesn't matter how tall you are, your body composition, or how much you weigh, if you aren't seeing yourself in a positive light and thinking good things about you, then none of it really matters, does it?

Your perception of yourself is something that often gets overlooked because of all life's external pressures, society tosses everything into a pressure cooker and it's up to you to take control of the mental and what matters to you.

How you think and feel about sugar is going to dictate how you deal with getting too much in your daily diet. The more knowledge you have about the harmful effects of processed added sugars, increases the likelihood that you are going to make more aggressive moves quicker to tone down and eventually vamoose the sugars.

Tips to Improve Mental

-Exercise regularly
-Read a book
-Meditate
-Try something new
-Go out with friends

-Make healthier food choices
-Do something nice for someone
-Do regular brain games like crosswords
-See your doctor and dentist regularly
-Get a new hobby
-Go dancing
-Take a vacation
-Have a bubble bath
-Take a half hour to yourself each day

Health Status

Your overall current physical and mental health status is a good predictor of your ability to get unhealthy sugars out of your diet successfully. If you are already suffering from health issues, like pre-diabetes, it's even more critical you take action to control your blood sugar levels now with healthy food choices and regular exercise to start.

If you suffer from depression, you may find it extremely difficult to get motivated to create new healthy habits, much less stick to them. Getting professional counselling and a full assessment from your doctor may be necessary before you can create a plan of action to blast sugar and get you healthy and happy.

You are important, and so is your health and happiness. Give yourself a break and take your mental and physical health status into consideration when looking to make any better wellness change.

Lifestyle factors

Your lifestyle factors influence all facets of health and wellness. If you choose to binge, drink, and party all night long, you're making it incredibly difficult to knock sugars out of your eating plan. The first cold hard one is that alcohol and alcoholic drinks are loaded with added sugars. Add to that how booze lets your guard down and when this happens social pressures usually squeak oodles of fatty sweet foods in.

Just ask any college student, drinker eat more junk!

If you smoke or do drugs, again you are tinkering with the chemical function of your brain and body, interfering not only in the internal processing and function of your body, but also in the food choices you make.

When less oxygen is getting to your major organs, and brain cells are lost, makes sense you're going to make Dumbo decisions when it comes to sugar party eating.

Clean up your lifestyle and your sugar-free, trim and sexy body WILL emerge.

My Thoughts...

I didn't get in too deep here, we are just looking to cover the basics, but it's very important you refocus regularly on the big picture of good health. All the factors necessary to get you to your fat loss goals, personal strength and agility goals, and new lifestyle factors you want to create that ensures you are healthy, happy physically, and mentally, and sugar-free till death do you part.

The ball's in your court, just make sure you never lose site of the net.

Chapter Eight - Additional V.I.P. Knowledge - Take Action

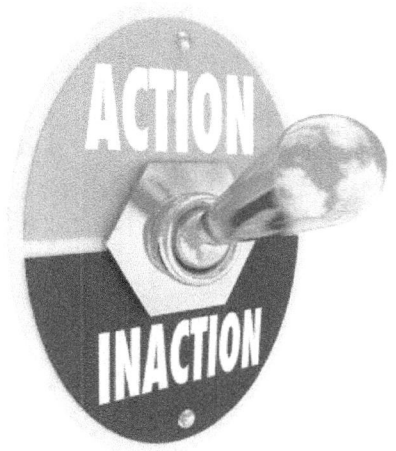

There are oodles of factors that will determine how successful you are in sending added sugar packing, losing pesky weight, and your overall ability to get healthy for life mind, body and soul, and make it absolute.

Let's have a gander at some key take action thoughts to set you up for success!

Exercise Take Action

Implementing regular bouts of interval training with both intense cardio and challenging muscle building exercises, core work, and stretching, is going to help you kick your processed food habits right out the door in exchange for a strong, toned, lean and super sexy body.

30 minutes to an hour of exercise every day is recommended for optimal health gain. This could be broken down into 30 minutes of rigorous cardiovascular activity 5-6 days a week, two or three sessions of weight training or strength training for 15 minutes each week, with core work and stretching every day. That gives you an idea of what you will want to work up to. Understand that anything is better than nothing, and if you can only fit in fifteen minutes one day, that's 15 minutes more than you would have done,

Cardio Ideas

*Running
*Jogging
*Power walking
*Hiking
*Biking
*Swimming
*Cross-Trainer
*Elliptical
*Tennis
*Boot camps
*Lawn trimming
*Skating
*Skiing
*Basketball
*Volleyball
*Soccer
*Squash

*Racquetball
*Skateboarding

Weight Training - Strength Training Ideas

*Gym weight lifting machines routine - upper body, lower body, and core
*Free weights at home or gym - upper body, lower body, and core
*Yoga
*Pilates
*Exercise bands for resistance training
*Exercise ball to add diversity and challenge to weight training and strength training
*Isometric strength training - using body resistance to build lean muscle

Note - stretching should occur before and after every training sessions religiously. The more you stretch and prepare your muscles to be challenged, the less change you have of tearing or ripping something that will sideline your for weeks or months at a time.

Hydration

Without water, you are good as dead. Water is actually the most essential element to your good health. It takes up more than two thirds of your body weight, and without it you would die in a couple days.

A few water facts...

*Your brain is about 95% water
*Your lungs are 90% water
*Your blood is around 80% water

Dehydrations kicks in when your total body water percentage drops below just 2%.

A car can't function without fuel and your body doesn't work without water, so drink up!

So, how can water help you with curbing your unhealthy packaged eating habits?

Ample water in your system is going to help flush harmful toxins from your system, this includes all the crap accumulated in your system from the sugars and sugary foods you've been munching on. Now, water can't get rid of all the extras your body doesn't need, but it helps.

The functions of water are:

*Lubrication- Water helps ensure everything from digestions and nutrient transports throughout your body needs water to catch air. The wet stuff helps lube up joints and tendons to ensure your mobility is optimal

*Temperature Regulation - Water helps to ensure you're not going to overhead by regulating your internal temperature. It's the water movement within your cellular structure that keeps everything in check.

*Toxic Removable - We already touched on this, water helps purge your body of harmful toxins built up over years. Urination and sweating are two methods where water aids in getting the bad stuff out!

*Nutrition Transport - Without water your body wouldn't have the ability to deliver essential nutrients to your internal systems for optimal system function.

You are physiologically dependant on water for great health. This means making sure you are getting clean and pure water into your system, 6-8 glasses a day minimum because this is one instance where you really can't overdo it.

Drink up the clear stuff to help diffuse your built up sugar stores and open the doors to fantastic health!

Better Food Choices

Here are a few ideas for better eating to help you chuck the junky stuff and slowly but surely get your eating picture perfect for you.

Instead of white bread...

Choose whole grain with the added value of nutrients and essential fiber.

Smart Move - A slice of white bread is approximately 80 calories with little to no nutrients. A slice of whole grain bread has the same number of calories, but loads of vital nutrients and essential fiber your body needs for optimal health

Instead of picking up cookies for a snack...

Choose whole grain wheat crackers or a piece of whole grain bread with a smear of jam or honey for that sweetness you're craving.

Smart Move - Just 2 small packaged cookies is about 150 calories, half of which is sugar. A piece of whole grain toast with a smear of jam is well under 100 calories, and you're getting nutrients and the fiber your body needs to feel full longer.

Instead of fruit juice beverage...

Choose a piece or whole fruit or fruit salad.

Smart Move - A glass of processed fruit juice can have up to 120 calories and 5 teaspoons of added sugar. An apple is approximately 50 calories with natural sugars, vitamins, and fiber.

Instead of having fried chicken and fries...

Choose a barbecued skinless chicken breast and a small baked sweet potato.

Smart Move - A piece of fried chicken and 1 cup of French fries can add up to over 500 calories and 25 grams of fat.

Instead of a restaurant serving of pasta with Alfredo sauce...

Choose whole grain pasta with tomato sauce.

Smart Move - 1.5 cups of pasta with cream sauce is over 450 calories. Creamy sauces are fatty are high in sugars. Cut over 250 calories by choosing a fiber rich whole grain pasta with lower calorie tomato sauce.

Instead of Fruitioo's breakfast cereal...

Choose whole grain cereal with little added sugar or large flake oatmeal with berries.

Smart Move - Refined breakfast cereals you see in those pretty boxes are loaded with added sugars, even the ones that claim to be "whole grain" and ' vitamin rich." Be VERY careful and read the label before you buy. A serving with milk is usually around 200 calories with a good dose of sugar. Your better bet is to have a bowl of oats made with milk, which has lots of essential vitamins and minerals, fiber, and very little sugar. Add some berries and you're getting protective antioxidants that help keep disease away, and a whole whack of flavor.

In time, you will learn how to make better food choices, just have a little bit of patience and understanding with yourself here. Commit to learning the nutrient components of the foods you love by reading the labels and recognizing there are oodles of "better" food choices out there for you. Ones that will help you kick the sugar habit, drop fat, gain energy, deter disease, and feel like a zillion bucks!

Accountability

This is a critical component of reaching your sugar zapping goals that often gets overlooked.

FACT - It's much tougher to give up when you have a cheering section. So many people have excellent intentions, but don't have the confidence and know-how to stick with new eating changes for the long run.

The goal here is to set your everyday environment up for success, and by having supports in place to encourage you forward, you're a hundred times more likely to reach your goals.

Having your doctor, a nutritionist and fitness trainer is ideal, but at least have friends and family there to help you stay focused and optimistic about kicking sugar out of your life for good.

Maybe you want to find a group of friends that want to commit to the same goal as you, people you can lean on when things aren't going so well, so you can persevere and win.

Possible Supports

*Doctor
*Nutritionist
*Alternative Medicine Specialist
*Counsellor
*Dietician
*Life Coach
*Psychologist
*Mental Health Specialist
*Family
*Friends
*Teacher
*Women's Group

My Thoughts...

Understanding removing sugar out of your life isn't a one shot deal is your first move. Next, by understanding all the external factors that influence what you eat, how much, and when, you are going to gain the control to conquer sugars.

Set yourself up for success and this issue you face today will soon be ancient history, TAKE ACTION!

Final Thoughts

You weren't born craving a chocolate bar or sweet chocolate cake, you *learned* to want it. Unknowingly, you
taught your mind and body to focus on sugar, desire it,
and crave more simply because you fed your body more.

Sound familiar?

Well now you understand just how harmful added sugar
is, not just because it makes you fat, but it also triggers
serious disease, zaps energy, and interferes with normal
optimal body function.

By creating a plan that works for you, a step by step ap-
proach to removing sugar from your diet, and replacing
the crappy food choices with healthy and nutritious ones,
you WILL succeed.

Use the knowledge you have gained from this book to
help you make better food and life choices for YOU.

If there is only one thing you remember from this, make it
that you give yourself time to get used to the healthier
changes you are making. It's not going to happen at the
snap of your fingers, but with patience, time, and perse-
verance, you WILL succeed.

If you make just one better food decision from reading my
words, then I'm a VERY happy writer!

In order for my books to rank and sell, they need positive reviews. If you enjoyed my book and have a few minutes to write a 3-5 line review about my book, that would really help me. Thank you :)

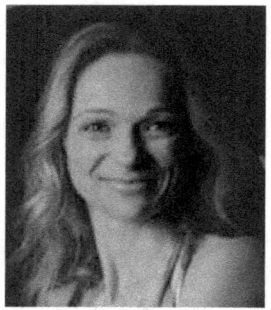

I hope that you enjoyed my book and you can check out all my other books by visiting my website at: www.flawlesscreativewriting.com

Disclaimer